Empower Your DNA: The Power of Vitamin C

Empower Your DNA: The Power of Vitamin C

J.Z. Parker

The Power of Vitamin C

Empower Your DNA

The Power of Vitamin C

Contents

The Power of Vitamin C

About the Author

J. Parker believes that each choice you make regarding your food lifestyle acts as either a deposit into or withdrawal from your "health banking" account. You can choose to make mostly savings deposits or check withdrawals. The balance of that account determines your energy, vitality, risk of disease, longevity, and ultimately the quality of your life.

J. Parker has worked in big food companies creating concepts. J.Z. is also a pseudonym. J. Parker, fondly referred to as J.P., writes to inspire a healthy relationship with food and exercise, along with practical tips to incorporate healthy living. And yes, he was a bartender at a point in time.

The Power of Vitamin C

Introduction: Vitamin C

Vitamin C is a very important vitamin in our system. It keeps you healthy. It keeps you young. It builds the fabric that secures senescence. Senescence means that you grow old slowly- so slow, it looks like you don't age at all.

You may think that you are getting vitamin C because you drink orange juice and eat an apple a week. The real question is- are you getting the right amount at the right frequency?

Vitamin C is a co-factor for enzymes. These are enzymes involved in the synthesis of collagen, carnitine, and norepinephrine, in the metabolism of tyrosine, and in the post translational modification of peptide hormones.

Vitamin C is a water-soluble antioxidant that protects low-density lipoproteins, and even cellular constituents, from oxidation. Therefore, vitamin C could reduce the impact of oxidant signaling, thereby affecting the likelihood of atrial fibrillation.

Whether you get something from this or not- Get this: Include vitamin C enriching foods in your diet or simply take Vitamin C daily. Get it from an orange or an apple or supplement. Your health and longevity depends on it. Some people take a combination (cocktail) of Vitamin C, Vitamin D3 and Zinc for good immune system.

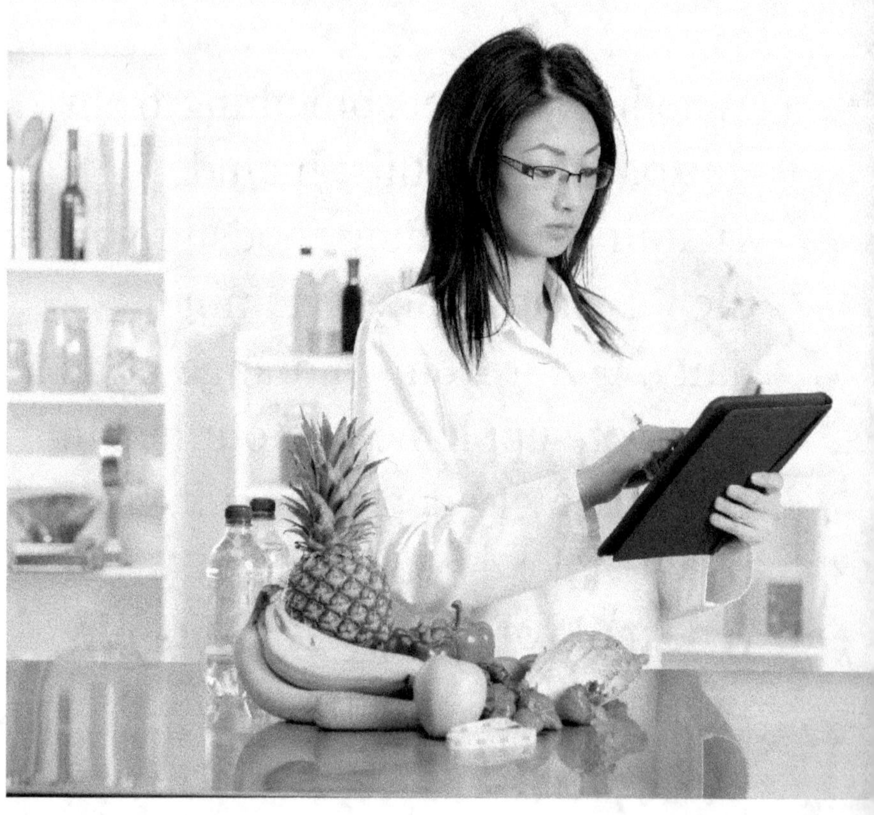

Jose is my friend. I knew him when he was a mover. It was a tedious work. He was strong, muscular and younger than Jim by over twenty-one years. Jim and I were his employees and we were just eighteen. Twenty something years later, Jose could not walk two blocks. Every step was calculated. Street bench was sought for wherever it might be located on the walkway just to rest the legs and the waist.

Going out to buy his favorite liquor was a hassle. When he tries to walk down to the store, his chest burns as if it was on fire. He complained of stinging pain in his limbs. The limbs become so painful and swollen that every step becomes an accomplishment.

The pain runs through to the waist. When he walks two blocks, his thoughts would be focused on how long it would take to get back to the house.

He wondered if it was now time for the dreaded wheelchair. For Jose's situation, he needed Vitamin C among other drugs not a wheelchair. His doctor confirmed it.

Jose's problems are peculiar with sailors, homeless people and sometimes prisoners. Jose was not a prisoner, sailor or homeless. These problems resonates with people who do not eat well.

Filling our stomach with junk food does not amount to eating right or eating well. Read my book *Eat*

Right, Be Happy. Jose also had bloody gums anytime he brushed. He had achy joints and back pains. He cannot walk two blocks because of pains.

When he laughs hard he gets dizzy. Ever heard of atrial fibrillation (a fib)? His eye doctor already told him that he will develop cataracts soon. He was getting worse. It is one organ complain today and two more the following years. He was falling apart. Jose is suffering from lack of Vitamin C and perhaps other supplements. He must see a doctor for diagnosis.

Jose was diagnosed with multiple deficiencies including vitamin C and D deficiencies. That was the diagnosis. He was placed on a heavy dose of Vitamin C for two weeks.

 The dose was later reduced to between 500mcg to no more than 1000mcg a day. Jose was also a smoker. When you are hungry, your body mechanism lets you know you want food. When you are full, your body mechanism informs you to stop eating.

Sometimes your body mechanism fails to work properly and you start having decreased appetite.

If only we can visualize what we put our bodies through. We punish our body so crudely and rudely, you may wonder in awe how your body takes all the punishment in stride. But like all things, the body has its thermodynamics and sooner than later, it succumbs to the laws of thermodynamics too.

Most people wake up in the mornings and dash off to the bathroom. They brush their teeth. They do the needed, take a shower and dress up for work.

On the road, they grab a cup of coffee with a choice of plain bagel or a cream cheese bagel or the choice of fried egg topped with cheese and tucked in between a choice of bread usually English muffin, croissant or two slice of wheat bread. This is breakfast.

For some people, breakfast happens on the go while in the car while driving. That is the breakfast routine for most working adults.

Later in the day, those same adults get a sandwich combo for lunch. Some may get pizza while others go into those locations where food is weighed/measured and paid for. It is also a routine. Sometimes, our routine becomes a routine that leads to ill-health and we do not know it. We just take things in stride sometimes because we do not know any better.

There are some people who because of time will make a cup of coffee as their regular breakfast. Sometimes, they will skip it entirely. Some may just snack on "something" until they get home for dinner.

You are now getting the picture. This routine is repeated everyday—day-in-day out for the whole year and the next and yet the next. Do you ever wonder why we are the most fed nation yet one of the least healthy?

How many times have you eaten ten servings of fruits and vegetable a day? You read that right. You are required to eat over ten servings a day. A healthy diet should include 10 portions of fruit and vegetables a day, doubling the five-a-day official advice, health experts have said.

A research, which involved a 12-year study, also found that vegetables were four times healthier than fruit.

The study, by University College London, found that eating large quantities of fruit and vegetables significantly lowered the risk of premature death. People who ate at least seven portions of fruit and vegetables each day were 42 per cent less likely to die from any cause. You may want to read my book *Bible Diet, An apple a day* book 1, 2 & 3.

Do you think the above eating habit can provide all the nutrients your body needs? The answer is an absolute NO! If this is just about vitamins, you can as well read it all on the web. This is about experiences with vitamins.

Some people will complain that when they brush their teeth, they bleed profusely. Same individual might likely complain of hurting limbs and unbearable pain in the joints. Suddenly, the pain progresses to the waist and walking becomes a fearful task.

When they manage to walk, they experience shortness of breath and they start looking around for the nearest street chairs to seat.

Soon, other symptoms accumulate; one piling on the other. The foot gets swollen from fluid retention (edema) and the skin is no longer smoothly layered as they use to be. The skin is now cracked and darkens in some spots.

To add to the frustration, you develop nosebleeds, your gum lacks collagen and your teeth gets loose in the gum. They are so loose, you feel they will fall out any day now.

You notice that little injuries starts to bleed for a very long period of time. You have lost the ability to blood clot fast enough.

You are getting from bad to worse so fast, you start to wonder. Meanwhile, your belly is getting bigger. Belly fat starts to grow fast. You start thinking you are eating too much; perhaps, you need to consider some exercises.

Nothing is working. So, it seems. Nothing is working because all the symptoms that has descended on your body are as a result of bad dieting, resulting in deficiency in Vitamins C, K and E.

The good news is that you have the supplements. Remember, it is called supplements. It were better if you get your vitamins from citrus fruits and juices, pineapples, cantaloupe, green peppers, broccoli and Brussel sprouts, tomatoes and cabbage; green leafy vegetables, potatoes and yams, cauliflower and asparagus, etc.

When you suffer pain, you know immediately. You even know the location where the pain is coming from. You take a pain killer. When you suffer fever, you know it and take prescriptions for it.

When you suffer nutritional deficiency, you cannot tell right away until it results into a problem.

Vitamins are one area of nutritional deficiency we think we understand but we don't.

We subconsciously compensate for this lack of knowledge by popping a variety of vitamins as we deem necessary. We feel mentally satisfied and then pop some more of the vitamins. If you take large amounts of vitamins as supplements, you may be setting yourself up for some trouble. You may poison yourself.

You may think that the Nutritional Recommended Daily Allowances (RDAs) are enough to guide people and help prevent vitamin deficiencies and side effects associated with large consumption of some vitamins.

What if your daily diet does not meet with the RDAs?

Simply put, though the RDAs are put in place to guide you, what if you notice some odd symptoms that you hardly can explain? In many instances, vitamin deficiency is the culprit.

What happens if you are deficient of these vitamins?

Signs of Vitamin Deficiency

If low in this Vitamin	Likely Signs of Deficiency
Vitamin A	Poor night vision; dry or cracked skin; dry mucous membranes from nose including the inside of the eyes; slow wound healing; damage to the nerves; reduced ability to taste, hear, and smell; inability to perspire; reduced resistance to respiratory infections
Vitamin C	Scurvy. Bleeding gums, loose teeth, gingivitis. Collagen is deteriorating, chronic low energy and strength. Chronic joint and limb is another symptom. Nosebleeds, skin rashes, slow wound healing, shortness of breath and

	many others
Vitamin D	Symptoms of bone pain and muscle weakness can mean a vitamin D deficiency. However, for some people, the symptoms are subtle. Even without symptoms, insufficient vitamin D can pose health risks. Low blood levels of the vitamin have been associated with the following: - Increased risk of death from cardiovascular disease - Cognitive impairment in older adults - Severe asthma in children - Cancer

The Power of Vitamin C

Vitamin E	The ability to absorb fat is lost. Welcome big belly fat.
Vitamin K	Blood fails to clot. Excessive bleeding.
Vitamin B1 Thiamin	Decreased appetite; weight loss; upset stomach; gastric upset (nausea, vomiting); mental depression; an inability to concentrate
Vitamin B2 Riboflavin	
Niacin	
Vitamin B6	
Folate	Anemia- being immature red blood cells. DNA cannot function as programmed. Symptoms include fatigue, headache, palpitations, diarrhea, as well as difficulty concentrating. There will be behavioral disorders and depression might also be seen in the person with

The Power of Vitamin C

	folate deficiency.
Vitamin B12	The lack of vitamin B-12 is characterized by abnormal walking especially in the elderly, memory loss, instability, depression, confusion, decreased reflexes, decreased hearing and abnormal growth in children. Permanent neurological damage can result.
Biotin	Anemia, irregular electrocardiographic activity of the heart, Dermatitis, Hyperesthesia and Paresthesia

The Power of Vitamin C

Vitamin C prevents a fib- yes, you read right. "Vitamin C- you ask?" You may say you've got to be kidding. Not only does it prevent the common cold and cancer, but it effectively prevents atrial fibrillation after cardiac surgery.

When some people laugh hard, they experience dizziness due to afib. Vitamin C is that good and important.

Some people have the impression that when you pop some kinds of vitamin supplements, it increases appetite. Increased appetite equals more food, therefore there is a fear of weight gain.

Although some people taking multi-vitamins report an increased appetite, there is very little scientific evidence to support that vitamins have any function in increasing appetite.

Deficiencies of many vitamins alone can cause a decreased appetite. So, in actuality, the feelings of increased hunger when taking vitamins may be due to previous deficiencies which when filled up when you drink the needed vitamins, means that the appetite returns to normal levels.

That you feel increased appetite than usual is an indicator that you are deficient in those vitamins.

Try vitamin C (ascorbic acid) of 500 mg to find out if you have an increased appetite.

Lots of people take vitamins to be healthier but may be concerned they may cause an increased appetite as they do not wish to gain weight.

Bear in mind that there is no evidence suggestive that this will actually happen. Even if any increase in appetite is noticed, it may be due to replacement of nutrients previously deficient, which is ideal for a healthier you.

 If you do experience a dramatic increase in appetite and it is ongoing, you should then contact your doctor to investigate the cause. Normally, when a deficiency is corrected, your appetite should return to normal.

The point of vitamins must not be lost to concerns of weight gain but to drive home the fact that vitamins play an important role in the body's metabolism and supplementation is required when indicated by low body levels. If deficiency continues over an extended period of time, it is possible that this may result in poor appetite and ultimately poor health.

Vitamin C and Scurvy

Scurvy can lead to sudden death if not diagnosed and remedied. Scurvy seldom occurs in the general population these days because of improved nutrition. However, the capacity for scurvy to slowly and silently destroy the organs are immense. When it starts with one organ, it piles up on to other organs. The effects of scurvy were well pronounced in the general population in the olden days.

Persons more likely to suffer from Scurvy are people with poor diet. Scurvy is a medical condition caused by a deficiency in vitamin C. It is also caused by malabsorption of this vitamin in the body even with that individual taking the recommended daily allowance.

Patients who are most susceptible to developing scurvy are infants who are weaned from breast milk, children who are picky with food, and people who are not getting enough vitamin C because of work or living conditions, such as sailors, prisoners, homeless individuals, etc.

Knowing the cause of an illness is not enough. The patient should also know the signs and symptoms so that he/she will know what to look out for in such cases

Symptoms of Scurvy Disease

The symptoms of scurvy are not limited to muscular weakness, joint pain, bruises, raised red marks by hair follicles and tooth pain while chewing.

The bruises and red marks are caused by hemorrhaging cells in the body while the pain while chewing is caused by loosening of the teeth and tooth structure.

There are a number of other signs but among the more noticeable are:

Sunken eyes

Internal bleeding

Gradual weakening

Muscle pain

Lethargy

Wounds fail to heal fast

Old wounds reappear
Tender gums

Pale skin

Liver spots

Loss of teeth
Pain in the joints

Generally, there are other symptoms such as diarrhea, fainting, and exhaustion.

One may start having trouble with the kidneys, lungs and other organ failures may set in.

1. Depression

2. Fever

3. Loss of appetite

4. Arthritis

5. Inability to gain weight

6. Black and blue spots on the legs and thighs

7. Partial mobility- walking becomes a hassle

8. Body aches

9. Swelling in the legs

10. Bleeding in the eyelids' lining

11. Slow healing of wounds

12. Enlarged joints

13. Anemia

14. Bleeding gums

15. Swollen gums

At this time you should have visited a doctor if you have not already done so.

How to Prevent Scurvy

The best way to prevent scurvy is to eat a healthy, balanced diet that contains plenty of fresh fruit and vegetables.

This will ensure that you have enough vitamin C in your body at all times.

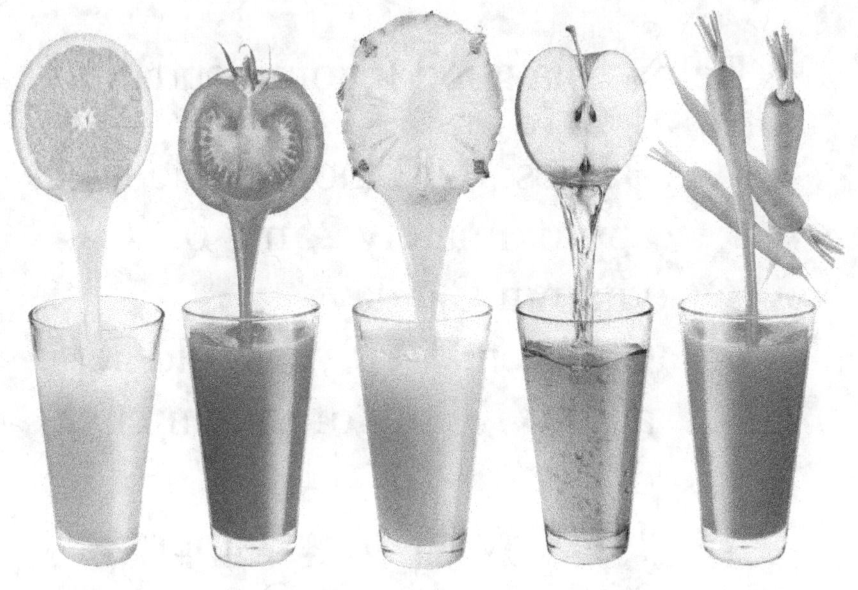

The Power of Vitamin C

Recommendations

Below is a good recommendation:

a. Babies: 0-12 months old—get approximately 25mg of vitamin C a day

b. Children: 1-10 years old get approx. 30mg of vitamin C a day

c. 11-14 years old get approx. 35mg of vitamin C a day

d. Other children and adults get approx. 40mg of vitamin C a day

e. pregnant women get 50mg of vitamin C a day

f. breastfeeding mothers get around 70-75mg of vitamin C a day

g. Smokers and heavy drinkers of alcohol may require slightly more

It is very easy for most people to get the recommended daily amount (RDA) of vitamin C from their daily diet. For example, eating one orange, a bowl of strawberries or a single kiwi fruit or an apple would provide you with more than enough vitamin C to meet your daily needs.

Consuming more than the amounts of vitamin C recommended above is not overly harmful. The only adverse effects you would experience if you were to regularly eat more than 1000mg of vitamin C a day (about 17 oranges) would be stomach pain, diarrhea and flatulence.

Sources of vitamin C

Fruit and vegetables are some of the best sources of vitamin C, including:

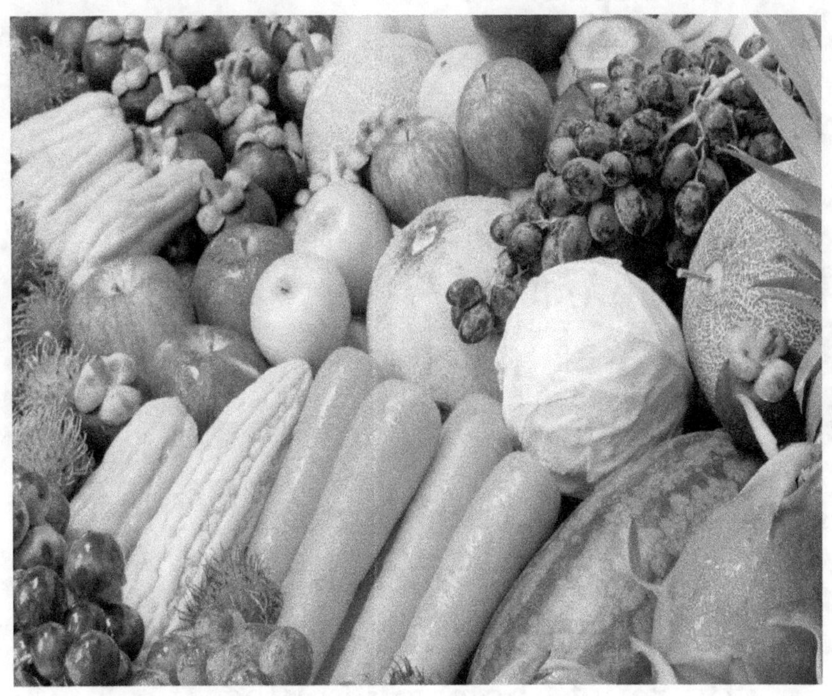

- Apples
- Oranges
- Lemons
- Limes
- Grapefruits
- Blackcurrants
- Strawberries
- Kiwi fruits

- Tomatoes
- Broccoli
- Asparagus
- Cabbage
- Green peppers
- Sprouts
- Sweet potatoes
- Etc.

It is much better to eat raw fruit and vegetables because vitamin C is easily destroyed during cooking. If you must cook vegetables, it is a better idea to steam rather than boiling. This is because vitamin C dissolves in water.

Levels of vitamin C also gradually reduce during storage, so frozen vegetables can have a higher vitamin C content than fresh vegetables that are left to stand for a long time in room temperature. A good example is pineapple.

Treating Scurvy (Scurvy affected mostly populations from the olden days)

The treatment is usually over 14 days. The deterioration of the organs may result in sudden death. Since sudden death may occur in patients with scurvy, ensuring adequate vitamin C replenishment in patients with vitamin C deficiency is the hallmark of therapy.

The restoration of body stores of vitamin C is very essential to achieving complete resolution of symptoms. In most adult patients, provision of 250 mg of vitamin C 4 times a day for 1 week aids in achieving this goal.

Identifying and treating comorbid nutritional deficiencies like iron deficiency anemia, folate deficiency and other vitamin deficiencies are the integral parts of managing scurvy. Provision of a balanced and liberal diet to meet the nutritional needs of the patient aids in recovery.

Scurvy is treated with vitamin C supplements, which can quickly improve your symptoms.

Some symptoms, such as joint pain, will usually resolve within 48 hours. Most people will make a full recovery within two weeks.

After alleviating your symptoms, you can notice the improvement. You must therefore learn good dieting habits.

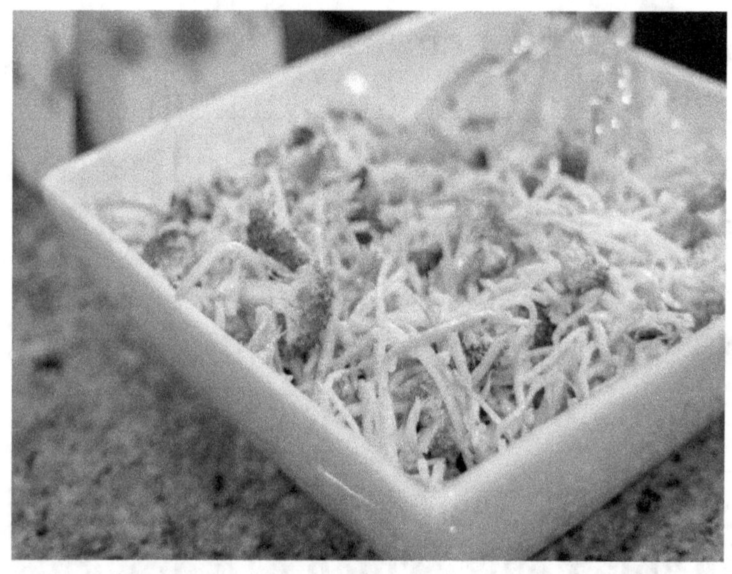

You should be able to get enough vitamin C by eating a healthy, balanced diet and you will no longer have to take supplements.

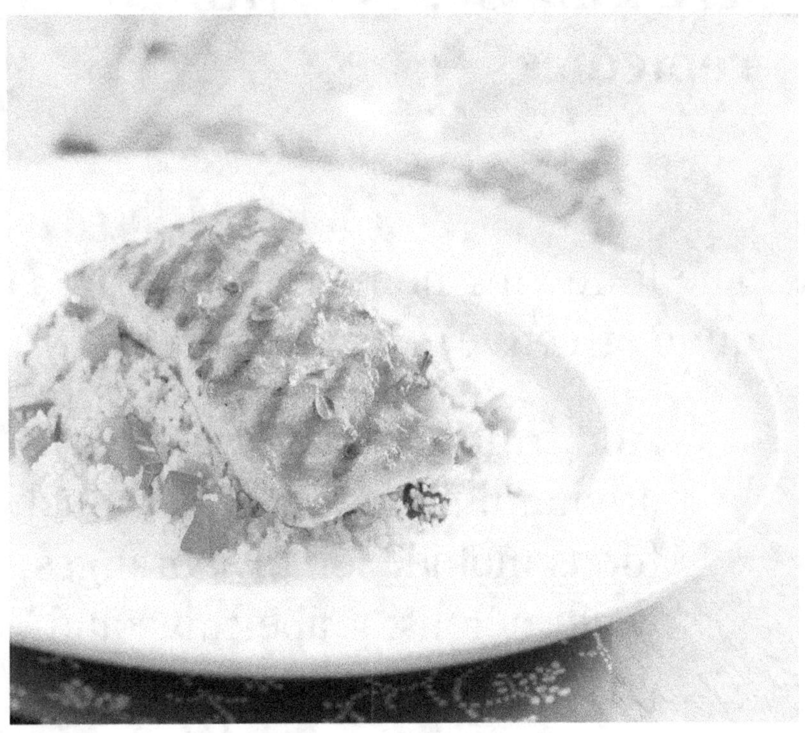

The Power of Vitamin C

Treating Scurvy with home remedies

The following home remedies are quite effective in treating scurvy:

- Add fruits and vegetables rich in vitamin C into the diet. Such foods include lemons, oranges, watermelons, grapefruits, and green, leafy vegetables.

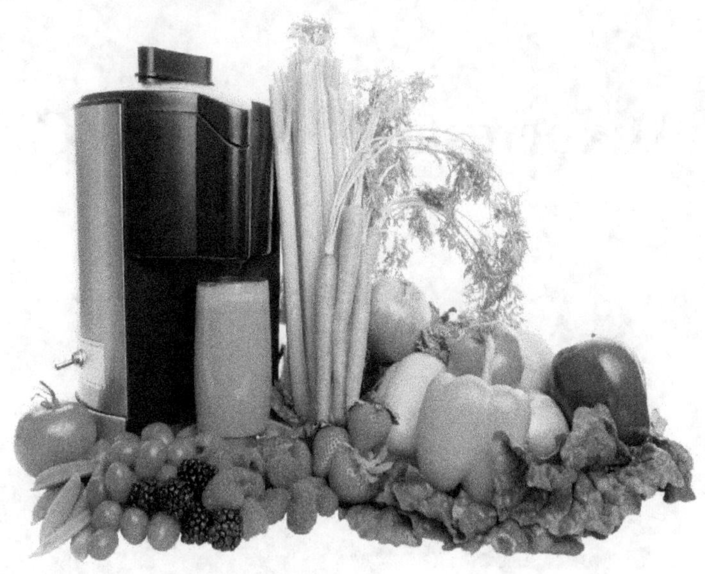

- Or an apple a day
- Add at least 100 g of spinach in the diet.
- Mix ½ tsp of powdered raw mango and 1 glass of water. Drink this.
- Drink a glass of fresh orange juice twice a day

Diabetes and Vitamin C

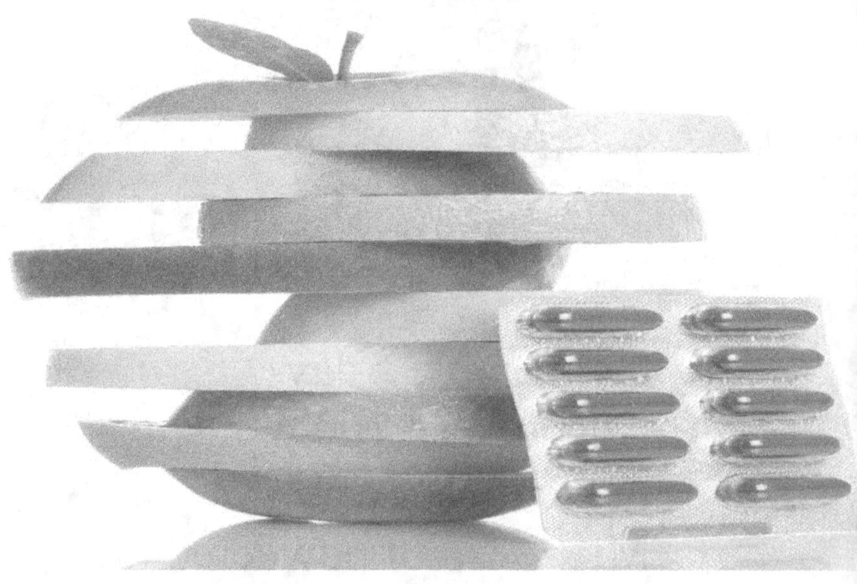

Have you ever wondered how vitamin C can help you if you are a diabetic? What about vitamin C and blood glucose monitoring and testing? Vitamin C is water-soluble. It has antioxidant properties.

There is a study on how antioxidants can decrease lipid peroxidation, LDL-cholesterol particles oxidation and improve endothelial function and endothelial-dependent vasodilatation – changes that lower the risk of cardiovascular disease.

In addition, current studies reveal that adults with blood sugar disorders and related complications tend to have lower plasma Vitamin C than healthy adults. All of this research strongly suggests that improving Vitamin C levels via diet and/or supplementation addresses an underlying cause of diabetes and its comorbidities.

Actually, an oxidative reaction occurs because of some factors such as high levels of your blood cholesterol, high levels of blood sugar, smoking, the surrounding pollution, and radiation. The free radicals will be generated in your body under the effects of all these factors.

As a consequence, several harmful chemical reactions are generated in your body, which lead to severe diseases like heart disease, arthritis, cancer, diabetes aggravation.

But, as everything in our body is balanced, here comes the role of antioxidants. In reality, the antioxidants are some body substances, which forbid (cut) the chain of further oxidation of these chemicals.

How it works- How antioxidants affect blood sugar levels

With regards to diabetics, due to uncontrolled blood sugar levels, these "bad" oxidation reactions are exceeded.

This is the exact moment when arteries clotting and heart disease and stroke will be precipitated; while death is one of their severest consequences.

So, the intake of vitamin C as an antioxidant is much recommended and scientifically proven in diabetics.

On the other hand, vitamin C gives a hand in the production of collagen—the type of protein that gives strength to your body bones, muscles, ligaments, cartilages, blood vessels and teeth.

Furthermore, vitamin C helps nitric acid action. Consequently, it can help you reduce the blood vessels spasms diminishing the risk for heart attacks and related heart diseases.

As a diabetic, you may face gum problems, muscles weakness, and difficulties in the healing of different wounds, especially skin ones. The intake of vitamin C can play a crucial role in reducing all these problems as well as the prevention of scurvy.

In addition, as a diabetic you can face other several diabetes complications in your kidneys, eyes and nerves. This is because of the accumulation of some substances in these organs of your body.

Vitamin C can interfere in the production of these substances, and practically, vitamin C can protect you from severe diabetes complications.

Smokers can benefit from vitamin C supplements and folic acid. These vitamins help the body fight toxic substances that invade the body due to the harmful and often deadly habit of smoking.

Alcoholics are likely to follow bad dieting habits. Alcoholics that follow poor dieting habits can benefit from daily supplements of vitamin C, thiamine (vitamin B1), pyridoxine (vitamin B6) and riboflavin (B2).

However, be very careful with any medicine. Do not believe everything you hear or read in advertisements and in various lifestyle magazines about multivitamins and or supplements.

Consult with your doctor before taking any medicine.

Most people without health problems do not need

multivitamins or supplements. If you are in any of these groups—suffering from a disease, vegetarian, pregnant or a smoker—you may need multivitamin supplements but ask your doctor first.

Do not forget that uncontrolled and excessive intake of vitamins can lead to dangerous medical conditions.

Conclusion

One cannot overstate the importance of vitamin C. Most of us take our bodies for granted forgetting that you are what you put inside your body. Some of us are only jolted to action after the body refuses to accept further punishment.

You give the body the attention it needs sometimes when it is too late. Vitamin C is very important in the nourishment of the body. Unfortunately, many people do not know they are not adequate in vitamin C.

Thanks to all the supersize this and king size that diets that are not particularly rich in vitamins but big in junk, carbohydrates and sugar.

Vitamin C intake is less than adequate in 20% to 30% of U.S. adults. This finding would probably apply to an even greater proportion of persons who develop atherosclerosis of such a severity to warrant coronary bypass surgery.

If 20 to 30 percent of Americans are deficient in vitamin C, one wonders the impact on the health care system because a lot of people will be suffering different ailments which ordinarily could just be prevented with the right dose of the vitamin C. Take your well-being and health in your own hands by practicing good dieting habits. Be healthy! Oh, by the way, Jose is back at work doing his moving business. Thanks to vitamin C.

Other Kindle books by this author are listed below.

1.

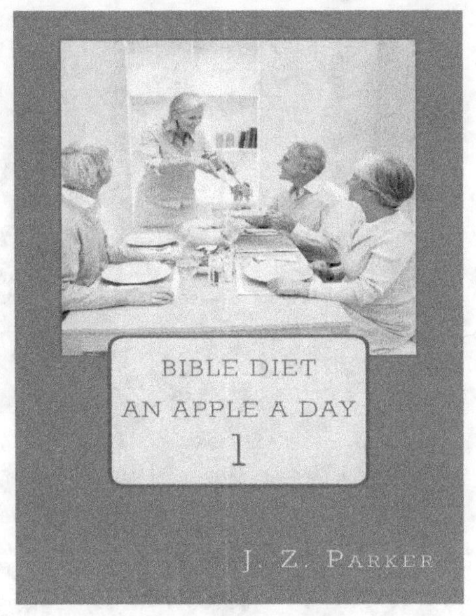

Gen 1:29 Then God said, "I give you every seed-bearing plant on the face of the whole earth and every tree that has fruit with seed in it. They will be yours for food. Gen 1:30 And to all the beasts of the earth and all the birds in the sky and all the creatures that move along the ground--everything that has the breath of life in it--I give every green plant for food." And it was so.

2.

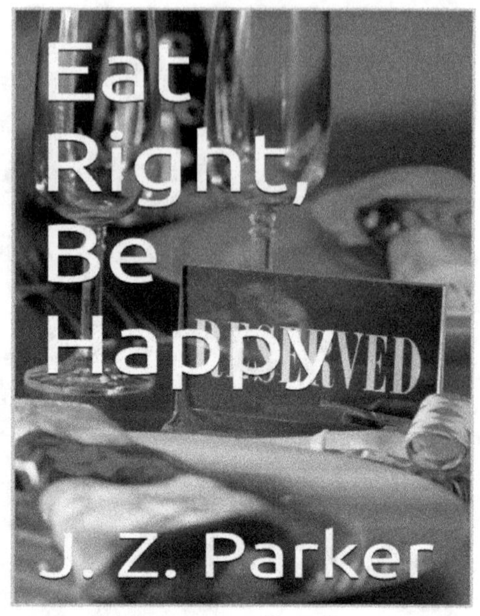

Most often, being overweight is as a result of incapacitation. Overweight is a direct result of damaged communication between the body and the brain.

To some overweight individuals, the reward is in the food at all times from beginning to when the last piece of the food is eaten. Any more food brought immediately will still have the same reward.

3. Quitting Smoking Easily:

For every cigarette you smoke, it reduces your life by 11 minutes. Thus each carton represents one day and a half of lost life. Every year you smoke a pack a day, you shorten your life by 2 months or 4 months if you are two packs a day smoker

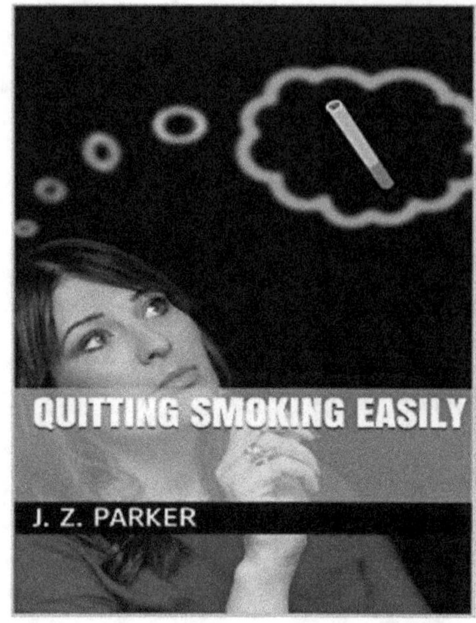
QUITTING SMOKING EASILY
J. Z. PARKER

Banana Blossoms: Banana Flowers:

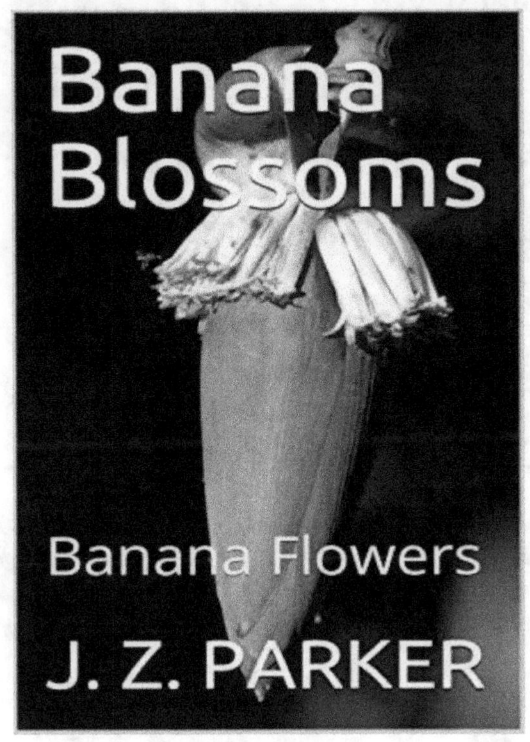

The most ignored and perhaps never eaten part of a banana tree, can reverse aging, diabetes and polycystic ovary syndrome (PCOS). There are so many other health benefits, so much so, you may wonder why we have not known about this part of a banana tree sooner. It has been a staple in most Asian countries. It can be prepared in many different ways in soups, stews, salads and sandwiches. This is one vegetable you need to eat regularly. It is worth it.

Good & Bad Plastics: Bisphenol A:

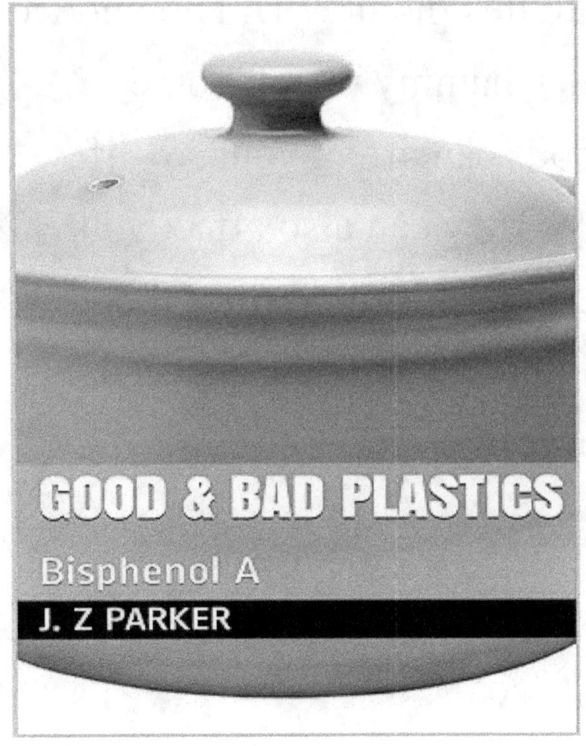

The wonder of canned food. Whip it open, heat it up in a plastic container and voilà, your meal is served. What is wrong with this picture? Did you notice the double whammy there? Some canned foods can affect your sex life negatively. They can also affect your libido negatively. How is your food stored? If you buy canned foods—any can—then read on.